Vision and Sight

Eye Care the Natural Way

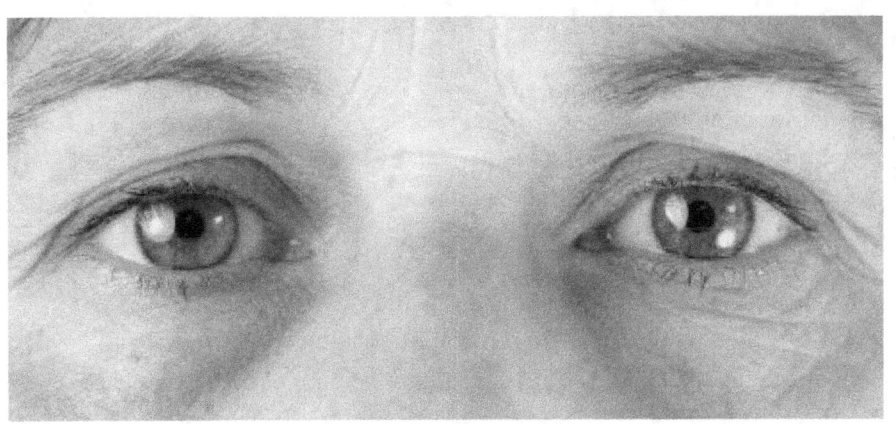

Science of Living Series

Dueep Jyot Singh

Mendon Cottage Books

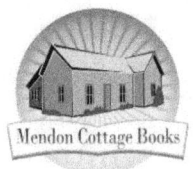

JD-Biz Publishing

Download Free Books!

http://MendonCottageBooks.com

Disclaimer

The information is this book is provided for informational purposes only. It is not intended to be used and medical advice or a substitute for proper medical treatment by a qualified health care provider. The information is believed to be accurate as presented based on research by the author.

The contents have not been evaluated by the U.S. Food and Drug Administration or any other Government or Health Organization and the contents in this book are not to be used to treat cure or prevent disease.

The author or publisher is not responsible for the use or safety of any diet, procedure or treatment mentioned in this book. The author or publisher is not responsible for errors or omissions that may exist.

Warning

The Book is for informational purposes only and before taking on any diet, treatment or medical procedure, it is recommended to consult with your primary health care provider.

Our books are available at

1. Amazon.com

2. Barnes and Noble

3. Itunes

4. Kobo

5. Smashwords

6. Google Play Books

Table of Contents

Introduction 5

Eye problem Symptoms 15

How Does Vision Work 18

Common Ailments Due To Age 20

Presbyopia 20

Glaucoma 20

Cataracts 20

Common Eye Ailments in Children 22

Myopia – Shortsightedness 23

Hypermetropia – Also Known As Hyperopia – Long Sightedness......24

Strabismus – crossed Eyes 24

Astigmatism 25

Amblyopia [Lazy Eye] 26

Eye Exercises 28

Palming 30

Index Finger Exercise 31

Tips and Techniques for Healthy Eyes 32

Proper Diet 32

Prevention tips... 33

Proper Reading Habits 35

Watching Television 36

Working on Your Computer 38

While Driving 40

Conclusion 43

Author Bio.. 48

Publisher.. 59

Introduction

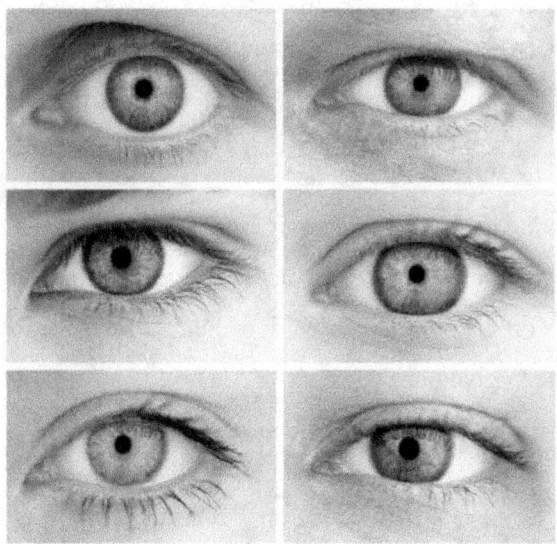

Eyes are one of the most precious gifts given to us by Mother Nature, but being human we have the tendency of neglecting them. That is because we have taken this gift for granted. This book is going to give you guidelines for keeping your eyes healthy, and full of vigor.

You may have read a large number of articles, in journals about eyes, and most of them are going to concentrate more about how you can beautify these windows to your soul. However, what is the use of all those artificial cosmetic enhancers, applied on your eyes, when you find your vision blurry, your eyes aching, and headaches brought about due to eyestrain?

Most of us tend to neglect the health of our eyes and take them, as I said for granted because we are so used to using them that we do not bother much about their general health. The moment they start aching, we rub them and go to the Internet to see for any remedies, which are going to stop them aching. And then we apply slices of cucumber or tea bags to those eyes, which are tired in a measure to refresh them.

Look at us, we have reached the stage when the eyes are strained and tired. Instead of shutting down that strenuous work before we reach that particular stage, we allow them to start aching, accompanied with headaches. Then we place ourselves on the nearest bed, with cucumber slices, teabags, ice packs, or anything else to give our eyes a bit of rest.

By the age of 40, we start finding ourselves confronted with vision problems. That is the time we are going to make our rounds of the ophthalmologist, and perhaps an eye specialist, who is going to tell us that we need corrective spectacles. We are either suffering from myopia – short sight- or hyperopia, – long sight.

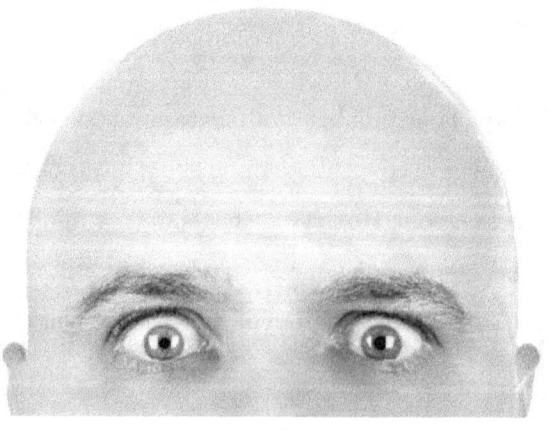

And then you put on your prescription glasses or perhaps contact lenses. And you remember to key in the number of that shop which sells you your glasses, on your cell phone because you do not know when you would need another pair and when.

The fact is that the care of our eyes and vision should have begun much earlier. Our eyes are our most precious assets, and looking after them could make the crucial difference between good eyesight and a blurred one.

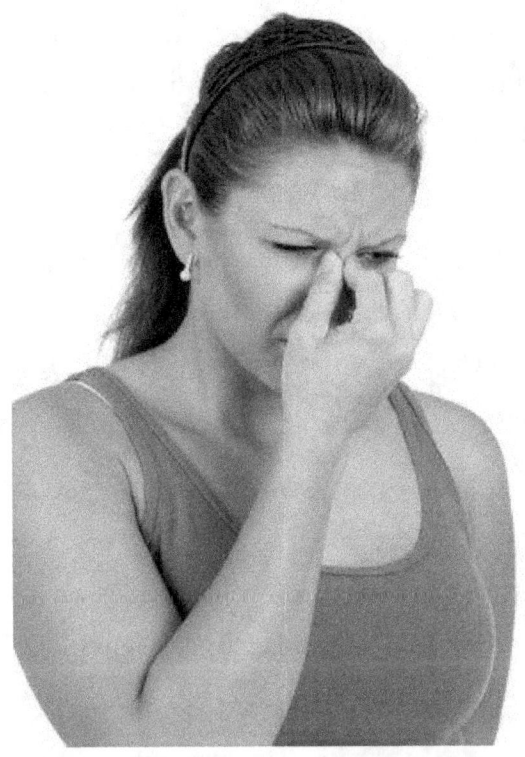

Tired eyes could be the reason for continuous nagging headaches.

The growing pollution, hectic and strenuous lifestyles, television, computers, bad reading habits, a dusty environment – all of these factors are going to add up to eye problems and just as we need to take care of our physical health, naturally, we need to take care of our eyes too.

I was about eight years old, when my teacher finally noticed that I could not see the blackboard from my seat, right at the back of the class. I was in the fourth standard. So I was told to sit right in front of the blackboard, cross-legged on the floor, so that I could write down the homework chalked out for the day.

But my teacher never told my parents that there was a possibility that I was suffering from hyperopia. I thought blurred vision was something natural and everybody suffered from it. It was only when my father told me to read a signpost about 15 feet away in the dusk and I said "what signpost," that he woke up to the fact that perhaps I needed glasses.

He had been transferred to a base about 480 miles away and we had gone by road as we did during all his transfers. It was my brother, who read out the signpost to "Donamalai", while I was still saying "what signpost", and even dad could not read the white letters in the dark.

We reached our destination at about 10:30 at night and were given accommodation in the guest house. The guesthouse was on top of a hill. After dinner, dad took my brother and I to the boundary of the guesthouse and pointed downwards. That was going to be our house in which we were going to shift within a couple of days.

What house, said I, squinting away in the darkness. Where?

"There, down there," said father, "cannot you see the boundary walls? They are painted white."

No. I answered still trying to decipher something out of the blurriness, and when he finally woke up to the fact that I was not joking, the first thing he did the next morning was to get me to the hospital and get my eyes checked.

He was shocked at the prescription number. I was badly hyperopic. And so I was fitted with huge pebble rimmed glasses at the age of eight with the prescription number of around +7.50 diopters.

That naturally colored the whole of my childhood because I was not allowed to play any games, for fear that I would break my glasses. The first thing I did in the morning was grope for them, because without them I could not see anything. I could see things clearly, if I held them closely in front of my eyes. But half a foot away, and whether it was there or not, all that was a blank slate to me.

The reason why my eyesight had deteriorated so much, during my childhood was because nobody stopped me from reading in bad light, especially when the rest of the family was asleep. I just put a cover over my head and continued reading The Golden Fleece, unabridged Classics, Lin Yutang[1] or The Adventures of Mungo Park with the help of a flashlight.[2]

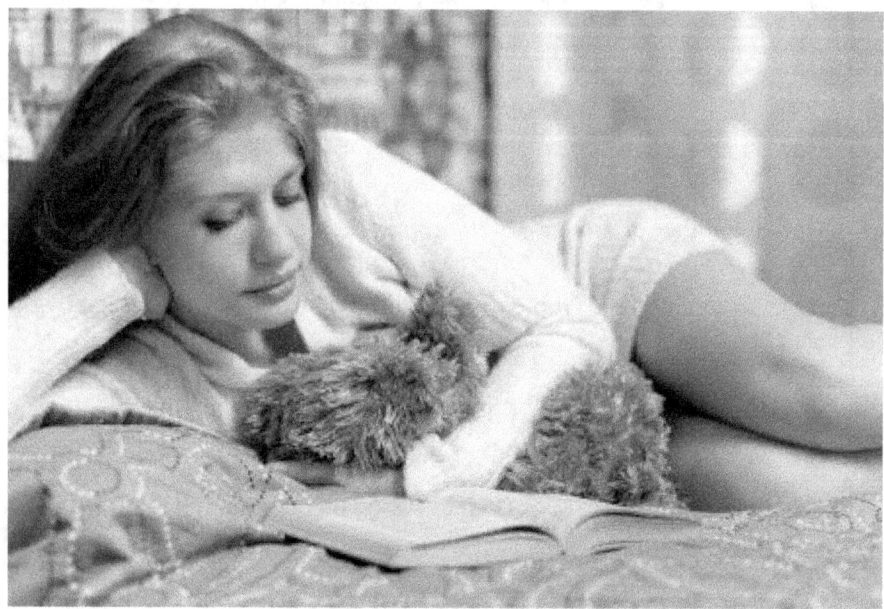

---

[1] I loved his List of Is This Not Happiness which included scratching one's back in the bath, looking at the moon and spitting out watermelon seeds, and hearing a cat pounce upon a most which has been disturbing your sleep in the night. This was what a child could appreciate fully, especially as we could relate to these points of happiness.

[2] Luckily nobody had told us that this was very advanced reading for a five or six years old, who were just given Heidi, and Grimm's fairytales as proper reading and suitable fare from the library.

And that is why by the age of five, my eyesight had started deteriorating a lot, because nobody could keep me away from books during the day or through the night. Luckily the house was full of books, including the now priceless Andrew Lang's fairy books because both my parents were great readers and when we were babies, dad read out from Shakespeare, aloud with us cuddled next to him.

By the age of four, it had become a challenge for us to recognize the place where he was reading in the book, and follow the words with our eyes. We did not understand half of the words, but we recognized the sound and pronunciation. And so we became confirmed book addicts.

That must have been very good for our own mental and intellectual growth and vocabulary, but it did not do much for our eye sights.

Luckily, my example and ruined eyesight made father look carefully at my brother and take care that he did not suffer from bad eyesight. He had 20/20 vision and still has it. So experience gained is always useful.

However, at that time there was this feeling that bad eyesight was inherited and that is why nobody bothered much about bad reading habits, especially in low light. So as father was hyperopic, it was expected that his first born would also be hyperopic!

So as long as I wore glasses, nobody bothered to correct my bad reading habits, especially lying down and reading, reading continuously without any letup and reading in bad light.

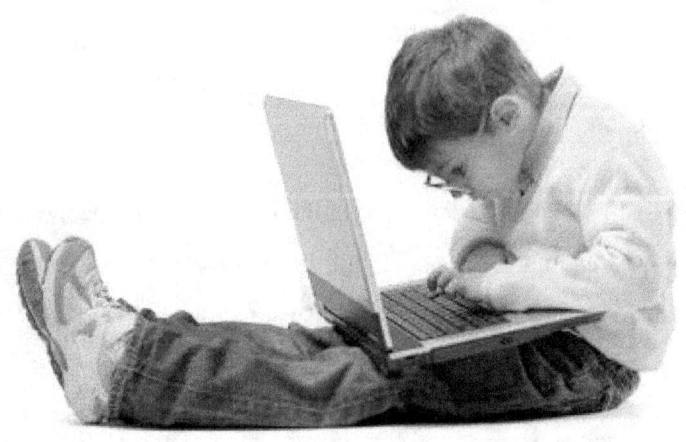

Is this what we are encouraging the next generation to be? Techno-geeks with bad sight, while they are still comparatively babies?

You need to remember that eye problems are not just connected with age. Children, like me, may also suffer from poor eyesight which needs to be corrected. A careful and intelligent parent should know how to look after children's eyes and care for them.

This bad eyesight contributed to poor performance in outdoor activities, especially games, so I had to compensate by becoming a complete hundred percent bookworm and Scholastic nerd. That was the only way in which I could gain self-confidence. Just imagine being the only student in the whole school with glasses on.

Even our teachers had 20/20 vision. And the problem with these glasses was that I suffered from headaches continuously, because of eyestrain.

Along with that, I was always referred to as Four Eyes or Owlet. I did not mind that much because I could retort with even worse nicknames for my tormentors, but for a sensitive child, it can make him feel inferior and even second-rate.

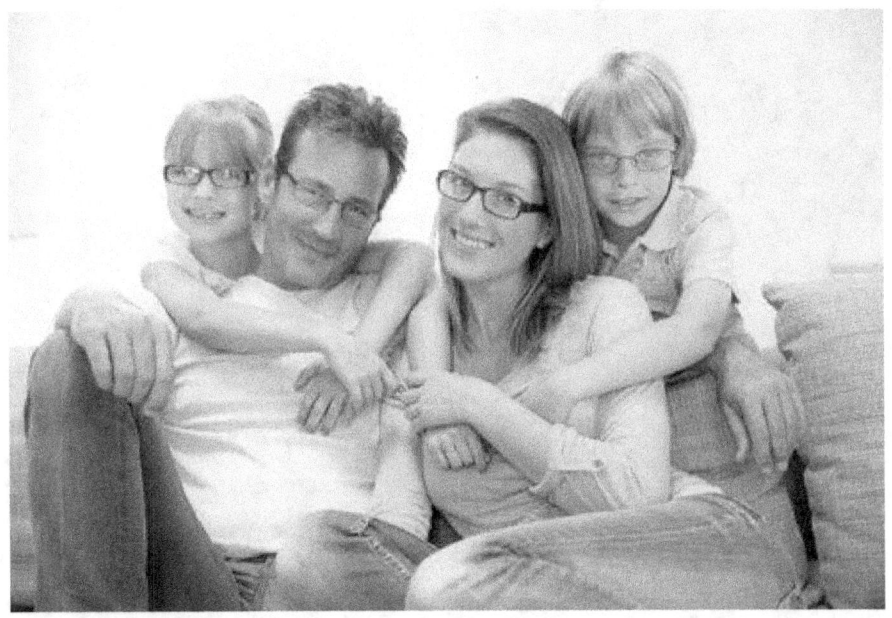

Glasses are so common among children today that parents have begun to consider them to be a part of life. During my school days they were definitely not common.

So, being an intelligent and sensible parent, here are the symptoms that you need to look out for, to make sure that your children are not suffering from potential eye problems.

Eye problem Symptoms

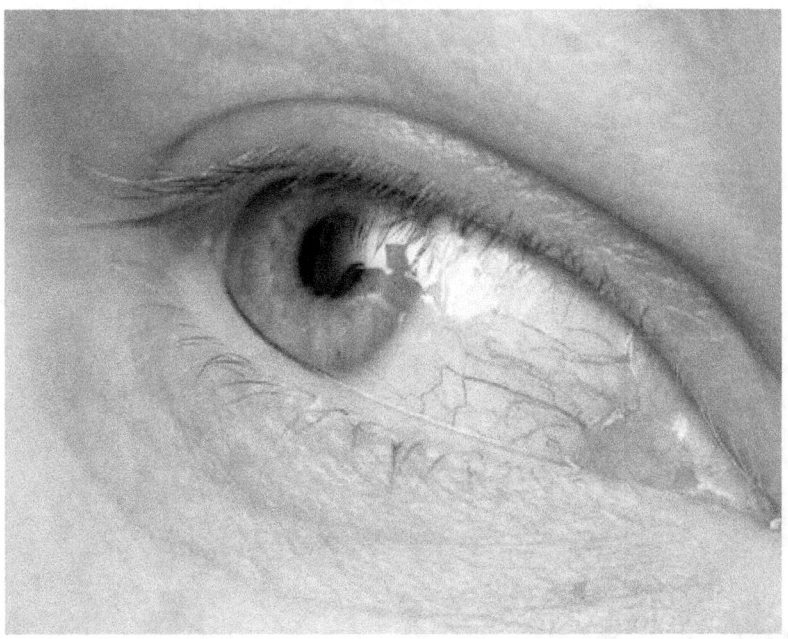

If you are over 40 and find it difficult to read your newspaper from the normal distance or when there is inadequate light, you may need glasses to correct your vision.

Even though my vision was corrected at the age of 24, with two operations of laser surgery, [+7.50 followed by +2.50] I still do not read the newspaper. I find the small print very painful. Even with reading glasses, I could not be bothered to read all about arson, abuse, terrorism, political hijacks, and maneuverings, and the latest idiotic antiques of the glitterati.

However, I put on reading glasses to read books or anything in print. This is because I found out that I was crinkling up my eyes and forehead to focus on the printed word, just to one – two feet away from me. This vision problem normally is connected with age, especially when you hit your 30s and 40s.

If you have been facing a blurring of vision or headaches, after doing some needlework or doing some reading, or perhaps after indulging in any other intricate work where vision comes into play, you may be facing vision problems.

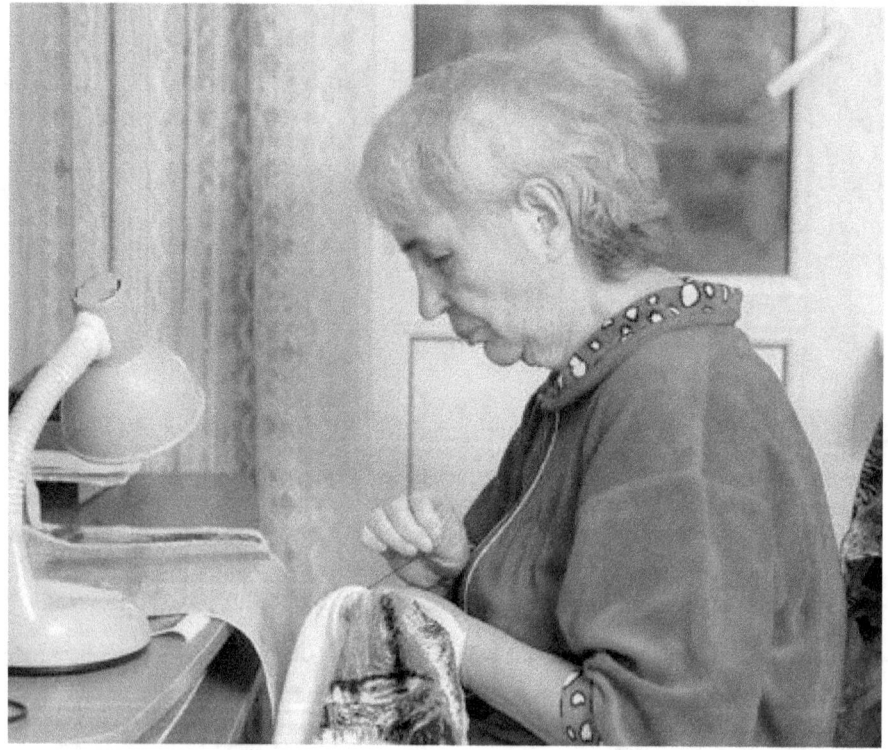

This lady is lucky. She has taken care of her vision throughout her life and that is why it has served her well in her old age.

If your child has not been able to see the blackboard clearly at school, and complains of frequent headaches, he could be in need of an immediate eye check. I remember my nephew when he was in the first grade. He came home with his folder empty every day, with absolutely no homework schedule written on it.

In our particular state, the children have to write out their own homework schedules even when they are in first grade. This gives them plenty of opportunity to learn how to write and also get accustomed to it.

My sister-in-law was horrified when he said that he could not see the board. She immediately got his eyes checked up and found to her great relief that his eyes were perfectly all right. It was only then she found out that his clear vision of the board was blocked by seven of his friends sitting in front of him!

After all of us, including the teacher had finished laughing, the little man was placed in the front seat, so that he had absolutely no excuse not to write down his daily homework in his folder!

Sensible parents place the television at a distance from where the children will watch. A number of parents could not be bothered about seeing that their children do not sit very close to the television. That is the reason why I have seen many children sitting about 1 foot or 2 feet away from the television, squinting away at the screen.

They are all potential prospective future patients for bad eyesight. If your child tends to watch the television at a closer range, it is possible that he is already suffering from bad eyesight. That means he cannot focus on the television screen from far away.

Watching television continuously for more than an hour is not healthy for your eyes, irrespective of whether you are a child or an adult. Whatever the distance between the television and the viewer should be at least 3 m (9 ft).

How Does Vision Work

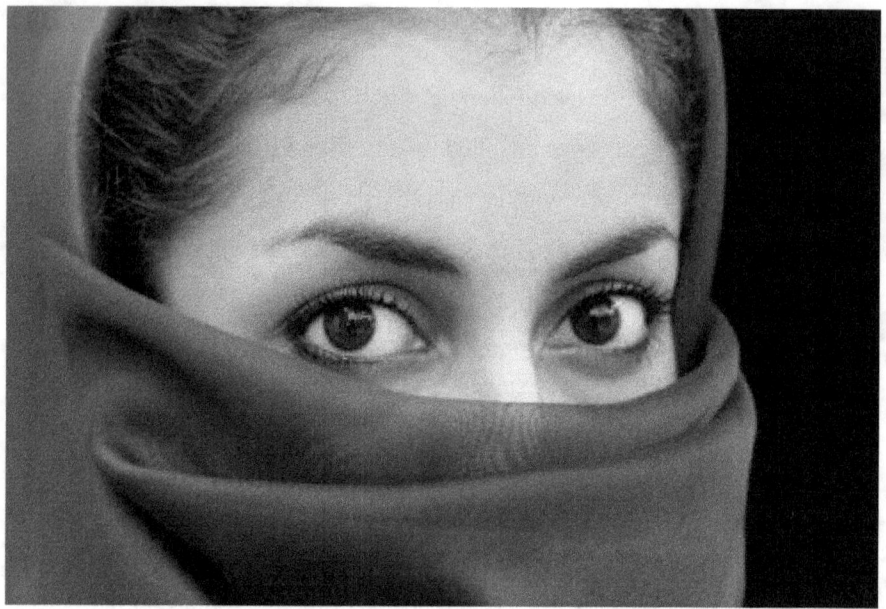

Your eyes may just measure about 2.5 cm in diameter, but they are your link to the world that contains all the beauty and colors imaginable gifted to you by nature.

When you focus upon an object, the light rays reflected from the surroundings around you are going to enter the eye. They are going to get focused through a lens. The image is formed at the back of the eye. This image travels up through an optic nerve and get stored in the brain. All of this is going to happen in nanoseconds.

And that is how you "see" the thing in front of you. However, when you are in the dark, because there is no light around you, to reflect and enter in your eye, you cannot see a thing. But the moment there is the faintest glimmer of light in the darkness, your eyes immediately get focused on that little light, trying to see your surroundings through the darkness.

Common Ailments Due To Age

As a person crosses the age of 40, several eye problems begin to occur due to the passage of time. These are the common ailments due to age, which can be found in a large percentage of us, possibly even before we hit 40.

Presbyopia

This is caused by the degreasing elasticity of the eye lenses. As you age, the elasticity of the lens in the eye reduces and the vision gets blurry. You may also find yourself suffering from headaches and eye fatigue.

Glaucoma

Glaucoma is caused by the increase of pressure inside the eyes. This eventually damages the optic nerve. This causes pain in the eyes, and if it is not detected in an early stage, it is going to cause permanent damage to the eyes. Glaucoma is considered to be hereditary in nature, although it could occur in people without any family history of this ailment.

Cataracts

Although cataracts normally occur after the age of 50, proper eye care and good health, could postpone it to a much later age. In cataracts, the eye lenses become clouded. This leads to blurred vision. The most common cure for cataracts is surgical operations.

CATARACT

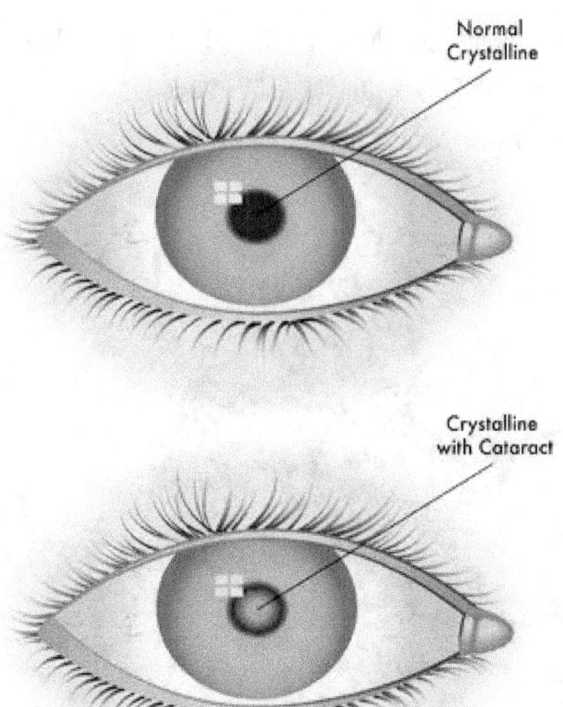

Normal
Crystalline

Crystalline
with Cataract

Common Eye Ailments in Children

What are the common problems associated with the child's eyesight? Well, there are some problems, which have been coming down the ages of which the nature is either hereditary or individual.

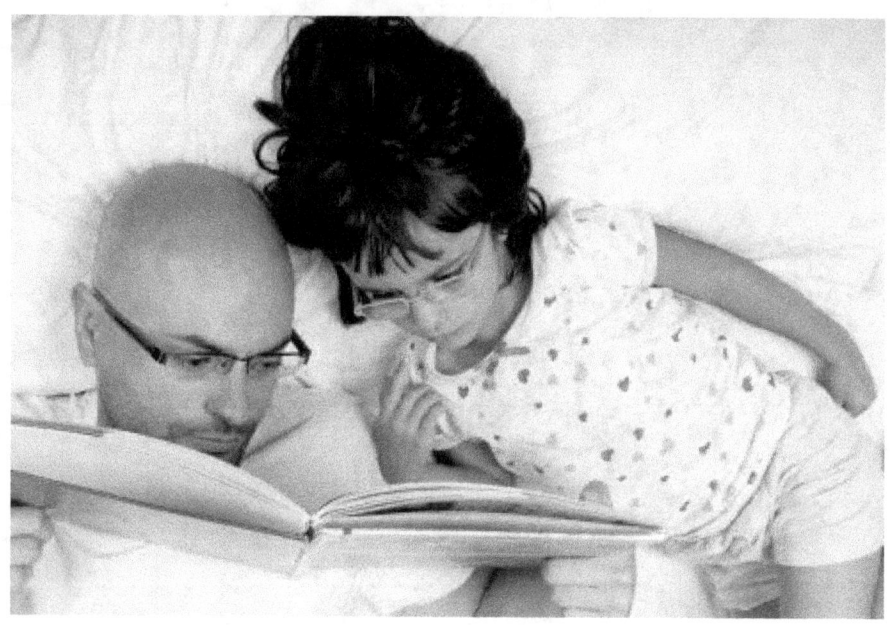

Reminds me so much of father and I, when I was a kid! Bad reading habits and thus the glasses!

The most common eyesight problems which are faced by children are:

Myopia – Shortsightedness

Just as in adults, children can also suffer from this problem, which makes it difficult to see objects that are at a close range. Distance vision however is going to remain quite efficient. While the child may have no problem seeing the television, he is going to find it a bit difficult to read. Myopia is usually hereditary in nature.

Hyperopia and Myopia

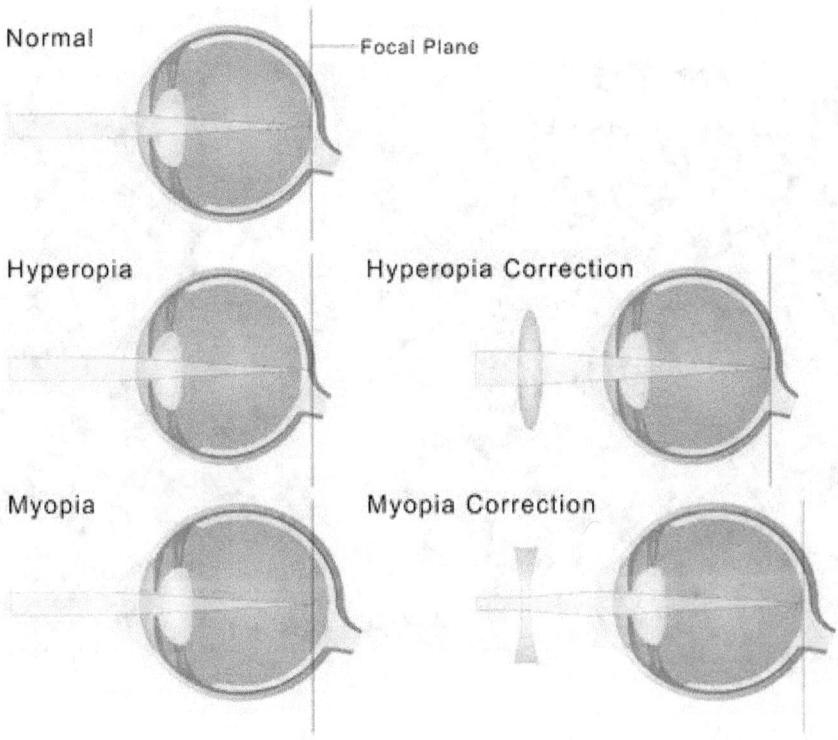

Hypermetropia – Also Known As Hyperopia – Long Sightedness

Contrary to myopia, this problem allows clear vision of close objects while the ones in the distance remain blurred. The result is that the child can read properly, but has problems watching the television or reading from the black board. The only drawback here is that the child is going to hold the book so close to his eyes in order to read, that he is going to suffer from tension headaches. Been there, seen that.

Strabismus – crossed Eyes

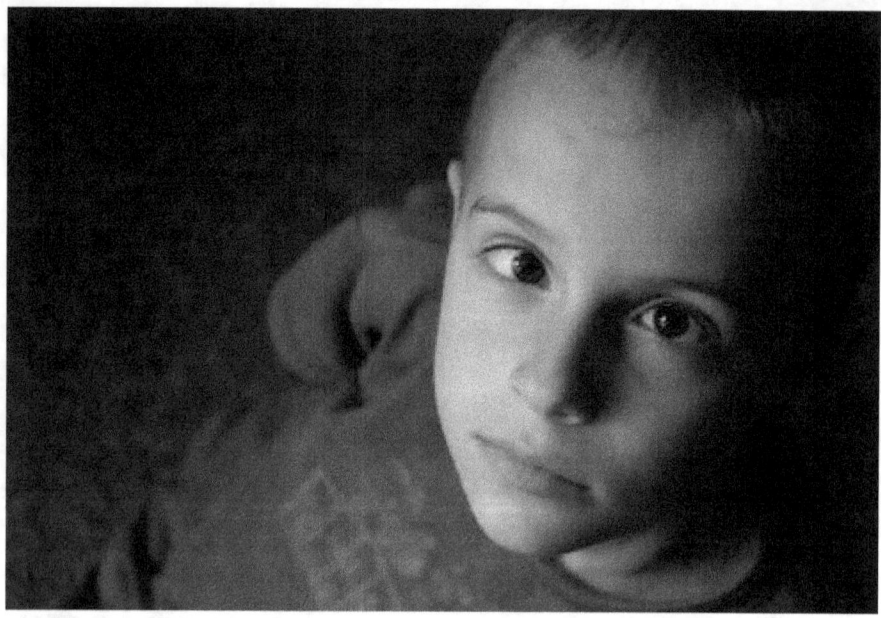

In this condition, the eyes are not properly aligned. The child finds it very difficult to focus on objects with both the eyes.

While one eye focuses on the object, the other eye is directed to the other side. This problem is easily corrected by the use of glasses and by eye exercises. When I was at University, I had a Junior friend who was suffering from strabismus. She was very good-natured and everybody liked her, but when we talked to her, we would find ourselves getting momentarily distracted by her squint. It made us feel taken aback for a second, before we got back to our state of normal equanimity and continued the discussion loud and clear.

She went for her holidays, and came back with her eyes operated upon. The squint was gone. There was this lovely pair of brown eyes looking straight at us, while we were talking and laughing. And the funny thing was that we kept waiting for her eye to squint!

Astigmatism

This results in difficulty of focusing on distant and close objects. This is going to lead to a lot of headaches, because you cannot see things near you clearly, and the same can be said for things far away from you. The basic problem lies in the uneven shaped corners in the eyes.

In some people, the outer transparent layer on the eye may have an uneven shape because of which the light rays entering the eye gets distorted. This causes blurred vision. Your ophthalmologist is going to recommend cylindrical lenses to correct this particular problem.

Healthy eye

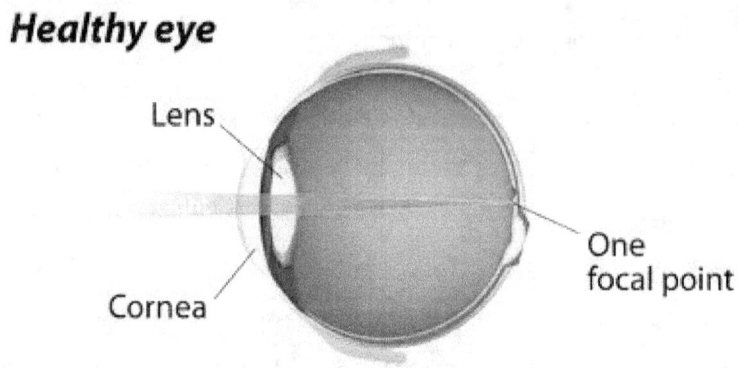

Lens

Cornea

One focal point

Astigmatism

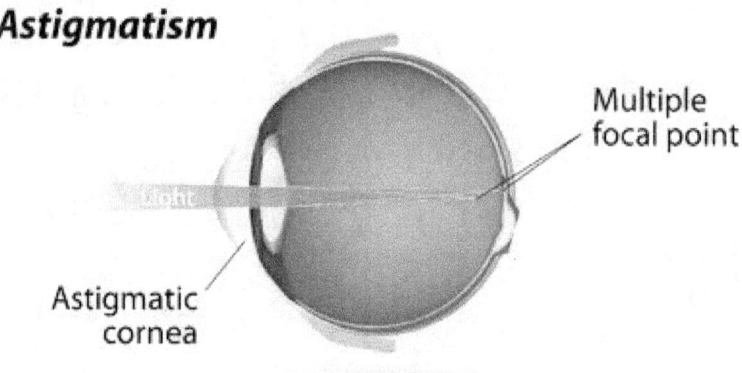

Multiple focal point

Astigmatic cornea

Amblyopia [Lazy Eye]

Sometimes the child has reduced central vision in one eye and lacks stereoscopic vision. That is when one eye keep ambling all over the place, when a child is trying to focus on an object. The problem can sometimes be a little difficult to diagnose, but a regular eye check could detect the problem so that it could be corrected at an early stage.

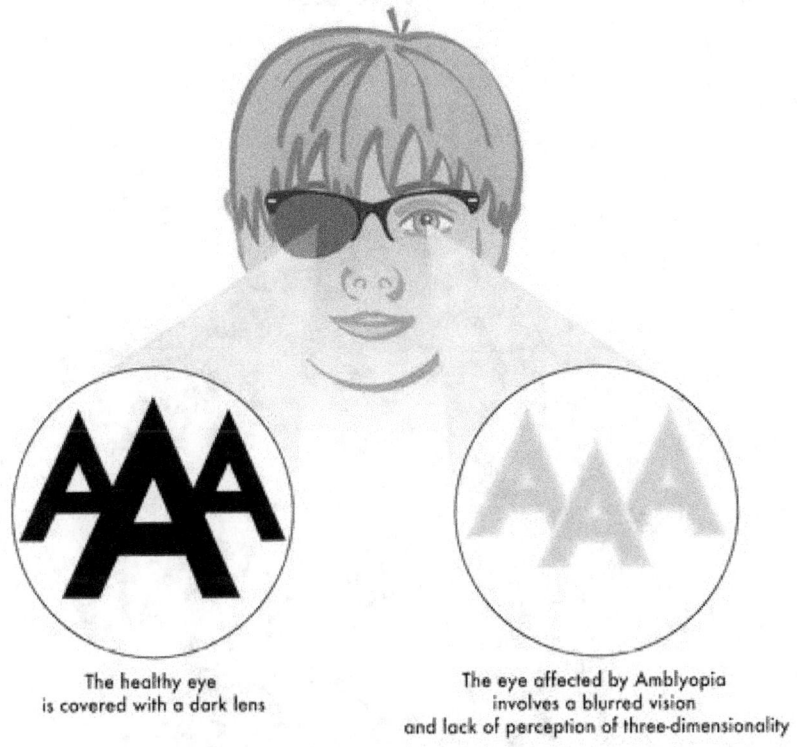

The healthy eye
is covered with a dark lens

The eye affected by Amblyopia
involves a blurred vision
and lack of perception of three-dimensionality

My grandmother used to talk about the way the elders in her ancestral town cure children suffering from lazy eye. They immediately put a black patch over the healthy eye. The child was thus forced to make use of his lazy eye more in order to focus on things. Within six months, the eye would be back to normal and would be a healthy eye. The patch would then be removed.

I think this is a very sensible method, because after all it is the eye muscles which need enough of exercise in order to start working properly and perfectly.

Eye Exercises

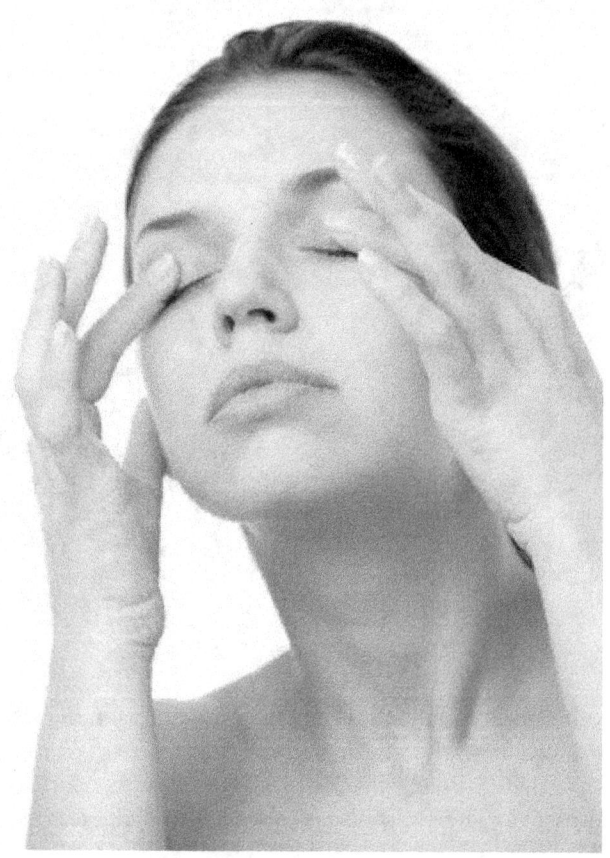

Even if a number of people have given the idea of high exercises plenty of bad publicity that they are not useful, well the answer is, they are beneficial. There are several eye exercises that are going to help in relieving eye stress. They also help in keeping the optic nerves and muscles in good shape. The bad publicity is given by all those people who do not have the self-discipline to do these exercises.

I remember an experience recounted by my grandmother. This was during the Second World War, when my grandfather was a Major serving with the British Army in Burma. He broke his eyeglasses. At that time, officers wearing glasses were allowed in the British Army, because I feel they were desperate for well experienced and war honed native officers.

He wrote my grandmother to send him another pair. The letter took about a fortnight to reach his home. By that time, he decided that he would try to get his myopic eyes back to normal by focusing on a newspaper, – guaranteed small print – by holding it near his eyes, and then a bit further away, to his eyes got used to that particular distance. He repeated this exercise every occasion he could get throughout the day.

By the time grandma managed to send him a pair of glasses, within a month, his eyes were healthy and strong, and he did not need those glasses at all. Until his death, 35 years later, he used glasses very rarely and never prescription eyeglasses.

So it is possible to get your eye muscles working properly again. My corrective surgery took place around 25 years ago, and with the passing of time, my eyesight has begun to deteriorate, yet once again. For all those people who are afraid that Lasik surgery to correct eyesight is good for a limited time period and the eyes go back to myopia or hypermetropia (farsighted) again, well, it has not happened for me these last 25 years.

However, like I said, my eyesight is rather blurry and not so clear, when I wake up in the morning, so the first thing I do is this particular eye exercise to get my vision back to "clear" again. Keep your head relaxed. Gently move your eyes from left to right focusing on the extreme ends. In fact I try to focus on my shoulder tips. Move the eyeballs from side to side.

Then start moving your eyes from top to bottom and focus on the highest as well as the lowest point without moving your head.

Now keep your head relaxed move your eyes in a clockwise manner rotating the eyeballs to the extremes. Next move your eyes in an anti-clockwise manner. Do all these exercises three times one after another. Then jump up from your bed, and start the day with cheer and enthusiasm.

Do this exercise routine, as often as you can, as long as you do not have an appreciative audience around, because possibly they are not going to understand the reason why you are squinting at them and making faces.

These exercises will help and relaxing as well as turning up your eye muscles.

Palming

When I was a little child, my father taught me this exercise in order to relax my eyes, when they were tired. I just had to cover them up with the palms of the hands in such a way that no pressure was spell on the eyeballs. When all light was cut off, he asked me to dream of something soothing, pleasant and nice like green forests, mountains, or anything else I liked to help relax me.

I found this exercise very pleasant! This helps relax the mind as well as the eyes.

Whenever we saw a really beautiful scenic vista, during our peripatetic travels and exploration, dad used to make us stand in front of it, and tell us to learn it by heart. After that we had to close our eyes and visualize it again in our "mind's eye". This was the vision brought up to mind, when we did palming to relax our minds and eyes.

Index Finger Exercise

Now this exercise is the one practiced by my grandfather in the experience recounted above. This is for the adjustment of the eyes to near and far objects for better vision.

You should do this when you are totally relaxed. Hold up your index finger – he used his newspaper – about 8 to 10 inches in front of your eyes. Now look across the finger at any object that is about 15 feet away. Repeat this exercise about two – three times.

My grandfather held the newspaper in front of his eyes, focused on the words and then slowly began moving the newspaper back, still trying to read the words. The eyes had to make an effort to focus on the words, in the initial stages but with the passing of time they got used to this particular exercise.

And within a month, he did not need his glasses at all.

This exercise helps you to focus on your finger which is near to you as well as the object which is far away from you. Thus you are exercising your eyes for total adjustment of both the distances.

Tips and Techniques for Healthy Eyes

Here are several measures that are going to help you keep your eyes healthy, till a late age. These are especially applicable to your children because they still have the rest of their lives to go through and healthy eyes are always an asset, especially when they are choosing particular professional fields where good eyesight is paramount.

Good nutrition correct habits and awareness can lead to better health of your eyes.

Proper Diet

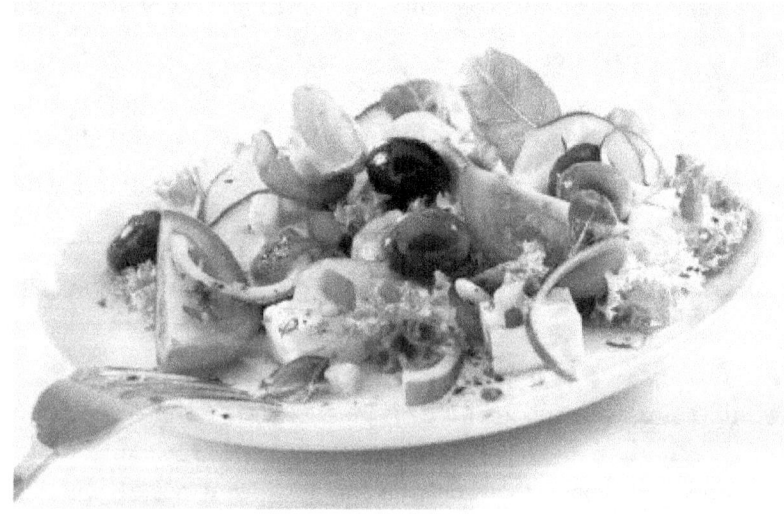

Green leafy vegetables, milk and a balanced diet, which includes lots of vitamins, minerals, and essential element are helpful in preventing potential eye problems. Milk, carrots, eggs, vegetables containing beta-carotene, and fresh fruit are all an essential part of a healthy diet to keep a growing child's body healthy.

Vitamin A is essential for good health and vision. Eating vegetables that contain this vitamin is known to prevent bad vision. Apart from this, calcium, carbohydrates, and proteins are also essential element which have to be included in your diet.

These are the foods which you need to include in your diet to get large quantities of vitamin A. Liver, tropical fruits, lettuce, dark leafy greens, dried apricots, bell peppers, fish, sweet potatoes, and winter squashes.

Prevention tips

Here are some common sense tips, which can help keep your eyes healthy.

- Avoid subjecting your eyes to dust, pollution and glare of the sun.

- Take care that chemicals do not find their way to the eyes. That is the reason any sort of harmful chemical product should be kept far away from the reach of kids.

- Do not allow children to play with sharp objects that may damage their eyes or cause accidents, leading to loss of eyesight.

When we were kids, father taught us archery with the help of traditional bows and arrows made by the tribal's living in the forests. The bow strings were made up of dried animal gut. The moment he handed us our bows, the first admonition was that if he ever saw us shooting an arrow anywhere near where a human being stood, he would immediately confiscate our new toys.

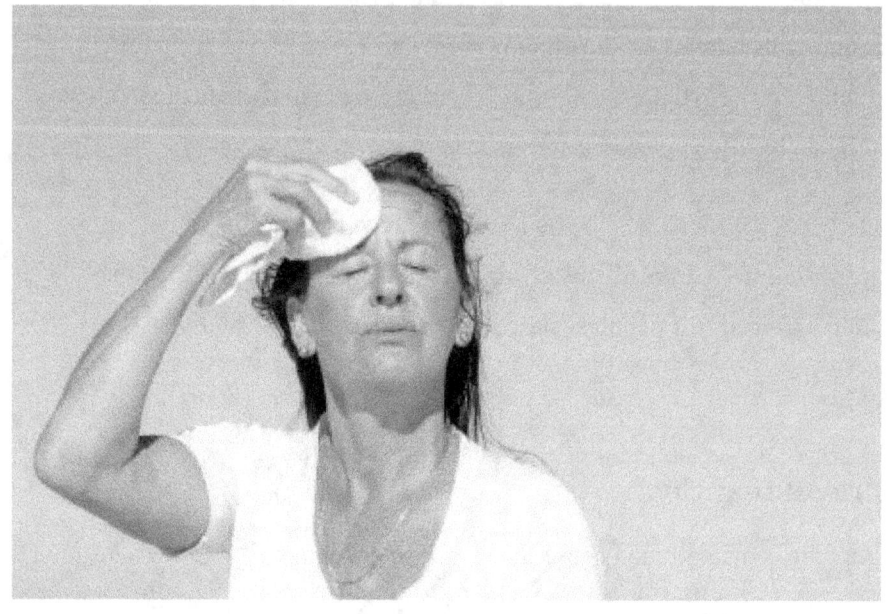

No sunglasses, no protective covering, or clothing, no hat, the lady is in trouble.

Our targets were always inanimate objects, far away from any human presence. When we asked him the reason why we were not allowed to shoot near or around humans, we were immediately given the example of King Harold of England during the battle of Hastings. Duke William of Normandy ordered his archers to shoot their arrows in the sky. The trajectory would bring the arrows down on the English army.

Even when common sense said otherwise, instinct always had human beings looking upwards to see the flight of the arrows and to see where they fell. And one hit Harold right in the eye, causing his death and the conquering of England in 1066.

And so we learned archery, without causing any sort of accidents of this sort ever.

Splashing your eyes with cold water relieves eye fatigue and freshens up your eyes. Remember to get your eyes checked regularly.

Proper Reading Habits

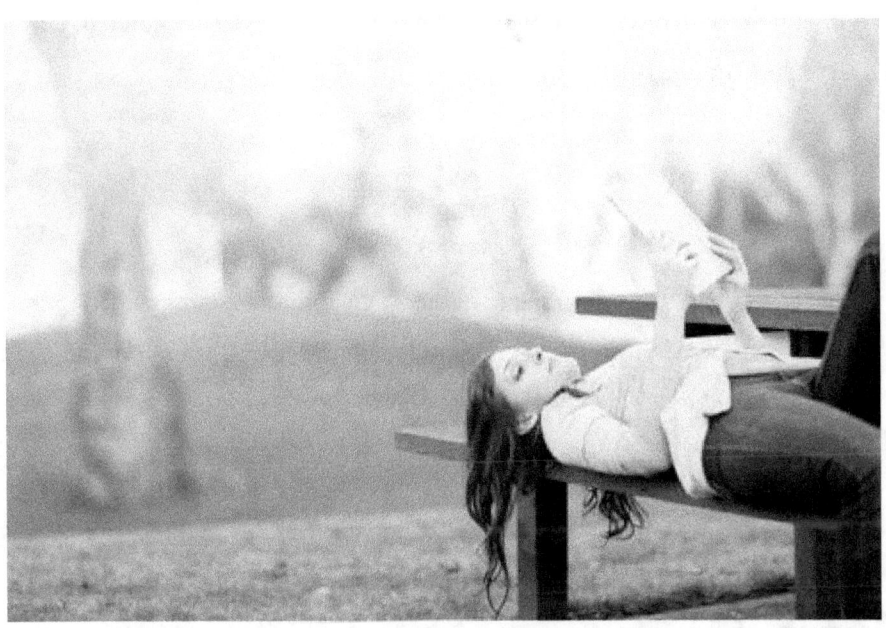

The distance is all right, but the position is wrong.

Good posture and healthy reading habits should be scrupulously followed, especially where children are concerned. Make sure that they do not read lying down. In this position, the eyes need to stress a bit more, when focusing on the printed word.

The correct distance of the reading material from the eyes should be at least 30 cm (1 foot). the back should be kept straight. Sagging down on the chair should be avoided.

Reading in a moving vehicle also is going to spend the eyes and should be avoided.

Always read in adequate lighting. The light should fall over your shoulder onto the printed word, so that it can reflect back from a bright surface onto your eye lens. Less light means that you will need to stress your eyes more, trying to focus on the printed word. That means your eyes are going to get stressed and tired easily.

Watching Television

I went to a friend's house a couple of days ago and found her grandson watching cartoons lying flat on his stomach on the carpet in front of the TV. His nose was about 50 cm (1 1/2 ft) away from the TV screen!

When I asked her why she allowed the youngster to spoil his eyes, she said that it was the job of his parents to discipline him and his mother – her daughter-in-law – did not brook any interference even from a grandmother, in matters of discipline.

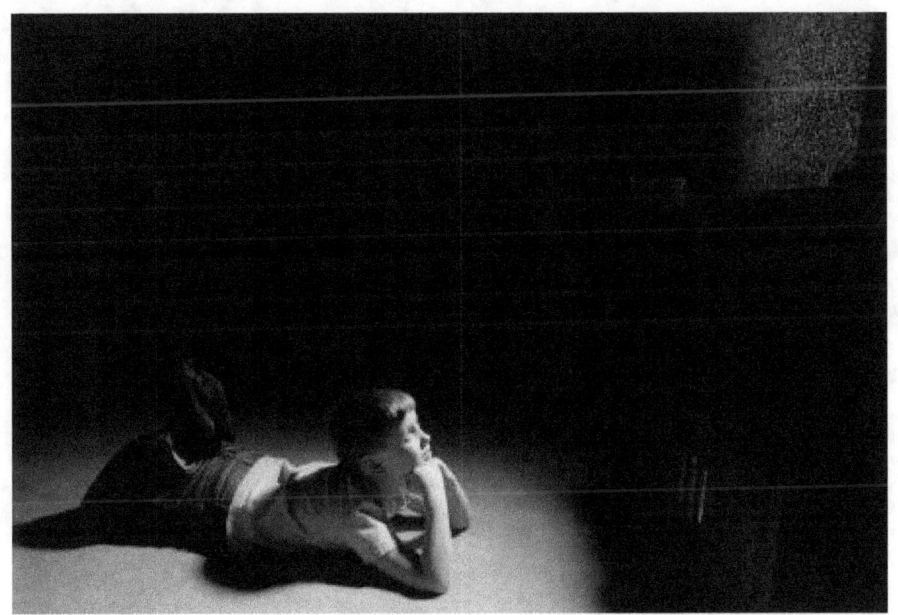

I kept my tongue between my teeth with difficulty. I knew what was going to happen to this little youngster just because his mother was a stubborn fool. He would soon be wearing glasses. By the age of three, he had already begun to squint and wrinkled his forehead, when looking at objects.

The correct distance between the television and the viewer should be at least 3 m. The posture while watching television should be erect. Many people tend to slouch or recline on sofas while watching the idiot box. This is an unhealthy habit. Not only is it bad for your posture, but it is also bad for your eyesight. You can place a support to the lower back which is going to help in maintaining the correct posture.

Do not watch TV for more than an hour. This same stubborn daughter-in-law had got her child addicted to cartoons, because she said that kept him quiet and out of her hair.

This child watched TV continuously for hours, staring at the screen without blinking. Blinking is necessary to keep your eyes healthy, especially when you are watching TV.

Watching television in a darkened room is also harmful for your eyes. You need to provide adequate lighting in the room. The light should preferably be situated at the back of the television at a higher point.

Working on Your Computer

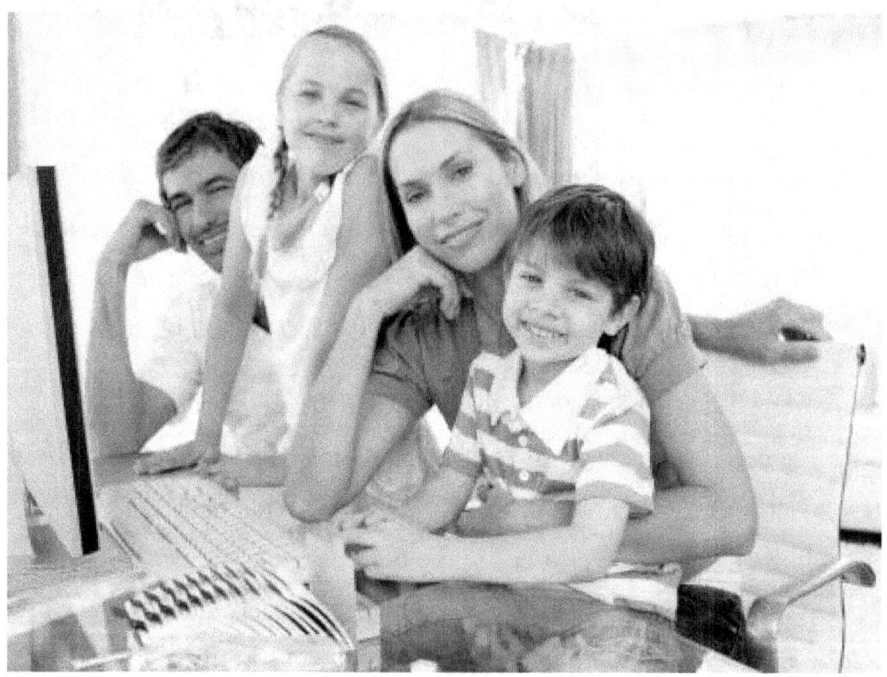

If you are working on a computer your eyes should be slightly above the center of the monitor. Make sure that you are sitting up straight in an erect posture, without any slouching. Both your feet should be on the floor. Your chair should have adequate support for your back.

Keep your mouse and your keyboard at the same level and close to your body. Do not rest your wrist on the keyboard when you are typing.

The latest operating systems in Microsoft come with speech dictation programs. Even though I have found them not so effective, or efficient as Dragon's NaturallySpeaking Professional software – which incidentally is very expensive, and thus affordable only by offices with a large budget! – you can manage to get away from continuous typing by dictating your messages through speech dictation.

Do not keep staring at your screen without blinking. Keep all your reading material near the monitor, if you are copying out something to be typed on your screen. When you move your eyes from the screen to the reading material, and vice versa move your head and not your eyes alone.

This exercise is going to prevent your neck muscles from getting stiff. I find it very useful especially when I am copying out files or information from hard copy for my future reference. This continuous moving of my head prevents possible spondylitis.

Adjust the monitor settings for better visibility. Now here is one trick, which I found out and which I do on whichever monitor I am sitting on.

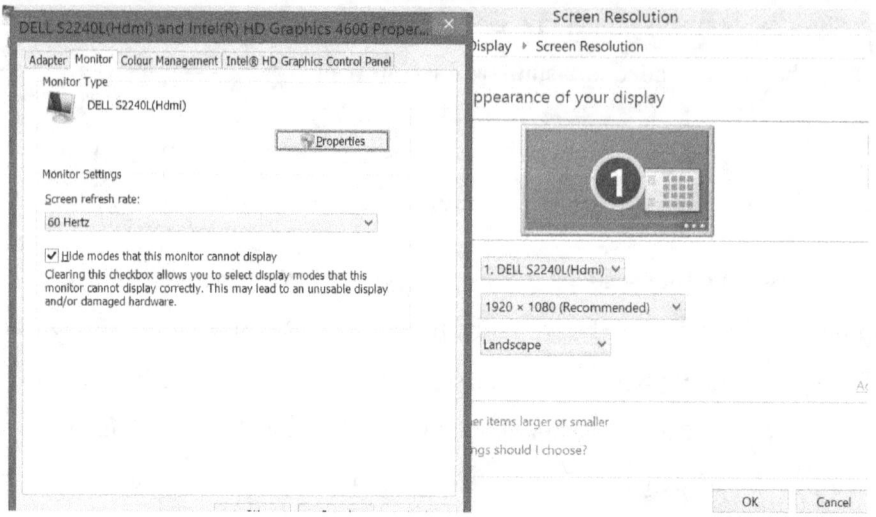

Go to the display properties of your particular computer. In the monitor tab, it is possible that you may have a number of display options like 60 hertz or more.

Control panel – appearance and personalization – Display [for Windows 8.1.]

Make sure the monitor screen refresh rate is the highest. Here it is 60 Hz and in some computers it is up to 75. The higher it is, you are going to find the screen even clearer.

While Driving

Use sunglasses while you are driving. These are useful in cutting out the ultraviolet rays of the sun. There also going to protect the eyes from dust and glare.

Avoid using darkened glasses without any sort of ultraviolet protection. These glasses dilate the pupil. They also allow more ultraviolet rays to pass through.

When I was still in my pebble rimmed spectacles stage, around 20 years of age, [I did not know about corrective surgery, then, nor was it well-known in our neck of the woods.], my uncle told me about prescription glasses which would turn into sunglasses. The moment I went into the sun, my clear glass lenses would slowly darken into dark sunglasses.

This was about 25 years ago, and I found them amazing, stylish, fashionable and cool. Notwithstanding the fact that these special eyeglasses were priced five times that of normal prescription glasses.

I still have them in my nostalgia box and the family still giggles at them, when they are taken out and displayed. The thick lenses were abominable, but as sunglasses, they were pretty hip.

I normally use antiglare glasses for night driving. These glasses cut off the harsh rays from the harsh headlights of the vehicles coming the other way. Once upon a time, there was a traffic rule in the country when all the headlights were half painted over with black paint so that the harsh headlights did not hit you headfirst. No pun intended.

However, people have managed to wriggle out of this particular rule for about a decade and now night driving is a torment and a peril. The latest jazzy snazzy models have ultra bright headlights which are touted as lighting up the darkest night and making it as bright as day. Never mind the drivers coming the other way and who normally have to put an elbow up against their eyes to protect them from the razzle-dazzle.

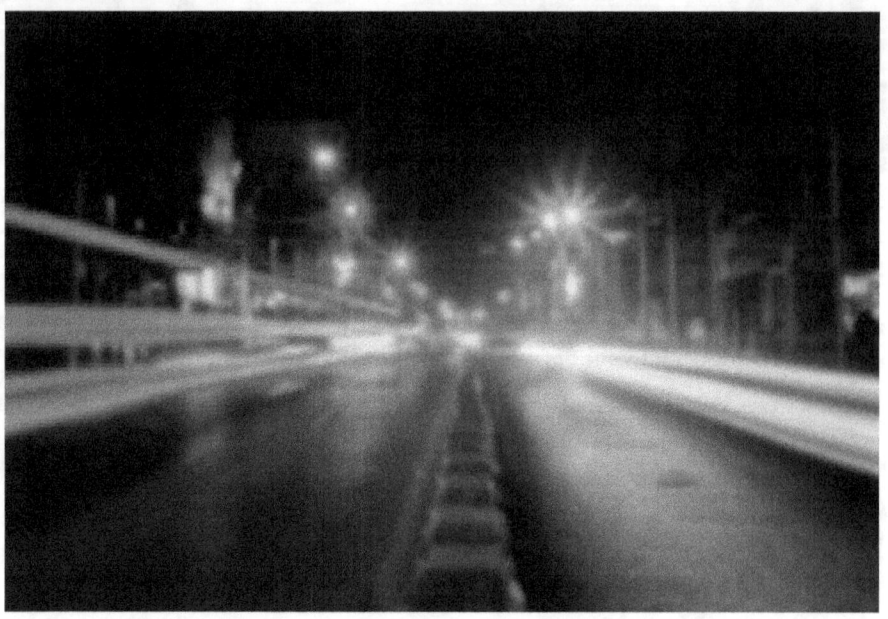

No wonder the statistics of nighttime accidents is one and a half times more than normal daytime accidents. But who listens?

Conclusion

This book has given you plenty of information about how you can take care of your eyes and protect them against damage. These rules and tips are common sense and time tested.

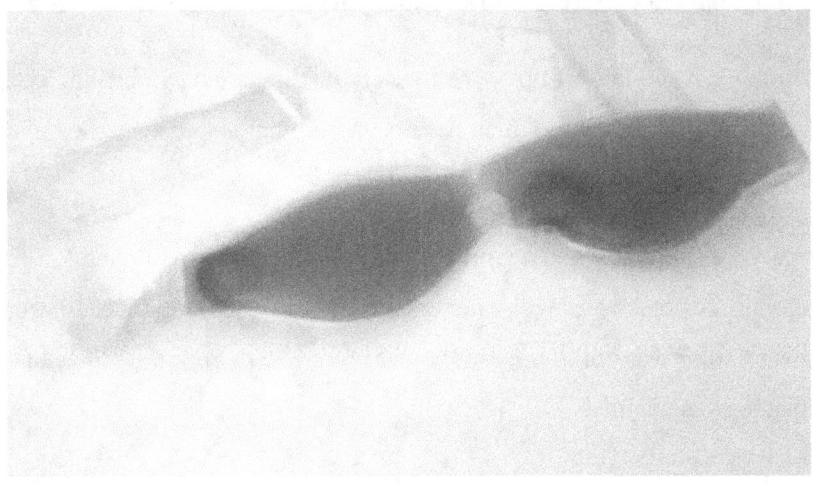

Here is another really useful thing I have found during my forays in Fairs and Exhibitions. I got it for about $1.20. I do not know whether it has made its presence felt on the Internet yet or not.

It is a Made in China gel pack, which looks like a pair of swimming goggles. You only have to put it in the refrigerator [not the freezer] for half an hour and it cools down to a really nice and icy temperature. After that, take it out and place it over your eyes and relax for 15 – 20 minutes until the room temperature brings the gel back to normal temperature.

At the moment, it is wrapped up around my forehead, cooling it, because the temperature is 35° outside! Very nice. It is fastened at the back of my head with Velcro.

So remember, all the guidelines and tips and techniques given in the book are going to help in keeping your eyes healthy for a long time. There is no reason why your most useful and beautiful assets should not serve you faithfully and without trouble throughout your life.

Just some last signing off tips, when we are talking about eye health. These are some natural remedies which have been helping people keep their eyes healthy down the millenniums.

Cataract was kept down to a minimum or prevented by mixing one teaspoonful of rosewater with one teaspoonful of fresh lime juice. 10 drops of this mixture was put in the eyes first thing in the morning. It stings but it keeps the eyes healthy.

When I was a child, somebody had told my grandmother that she could cure my eyes by putting the fresh dew off rose petals in my eyes at Dawn. I still fondly remember my much loved grandmother waking me up early in the morning so that she could put those dew drops in my eyes and then tell me to go back to sleep again.

I do not think those dew drops improved the health of my eyes with weak muscles, but they kept my eyes clean! I still remember this caring action with such fondness. Even though I did not appreciate it at that time, especially when one was subjected to fresh icy cold dew drops in the winter!

If your eyes are burning, all you have to do is mash one banana, along with a little bit of yogurt and water. Eat this twice a day and your eyes will stop burning.

Also, grind an onion with a teaspoonful of black pepper and poppy seeds which have been soaked in half a cup of milk. Poppy seeds are normally soaked overnight in the milk for natural herbal preparations in the East. According to the medicine men, this milk adds to the potency and power of poppy seeds, which incidentally are obtained from the same flower which gives you opium.

Apply this paste on your head, especially your forehead area. That is because in ancient times any sort of burning sensation in the eyes was supposed to be heat in the head area which had to be cooled down. Allow it to dry in 20 minutes and wash with warm water.

Suffering from eyestrain? All you have to do is boil half a teaspoonful of fennel seeds in a cup of water and delete is reduced to half. Cool it down and you can use this as eye drops as long as there is no fear of contamination.

This is a remedy I have been giving all my friends who suffer from dark circles around their eyes. I cannot do anything about their hectic lifestyles, and paucity of eight hours sleep every day. So to reduce the dark circles they need to drink tomato juice with a few mint leaves and a little lemon juice and salt to detoxify their bodies.

They should also soak cotton wool in cucumber or potato juice and apply it around the eyes. They are going to see a change within two – three weeks.

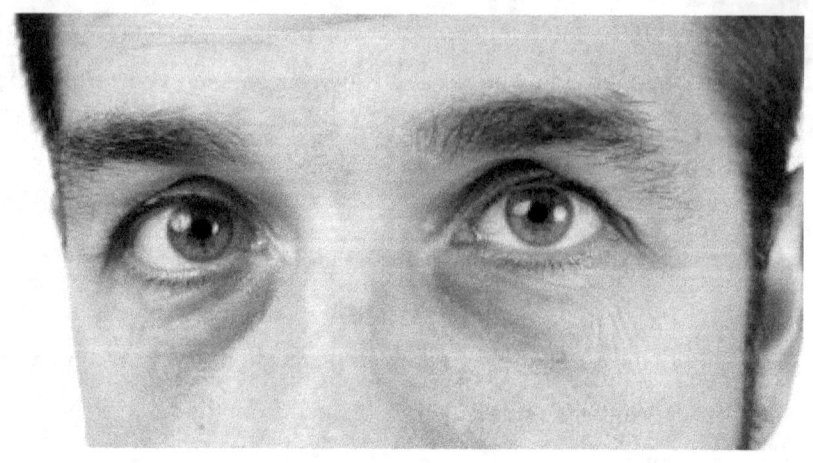

Dark circles can be health related, fatigue related, and even environment related, especially in highly polluted areas.

Another natural dark circle removal remedy is made with 1 teaspoon tomato juice, half a teaspoonful of lemon juice, a pinch of turmeric powder and a little oatmeal or bran or chickpea flour. Make a paste of this and apply in the affected areas. Leave for 10 minutes and wash off with warm water.

Tired eyes can be refreshed by adding a drop of lavender oil to 500 mL [2 ½ cups] of water. Shake the solution well dip to cotton wool pads in the liquid. Squeeze out the excess water and place one pad over each eye. If you wear contact lenses remove them before you do this relaxing activity.

A friend told me this remedy for weak eyes. Remove the seeds from a small green cardamom. Mix the seeds up with 1 tablespoon full of honey and lick the spoon, first thing every morning on an empty stomach. This freshly prepared remedy, every morning, is supposed to strengthen the eyes.

Try it out. If only for the chance to lick a tablespoonful of honey in the morning!

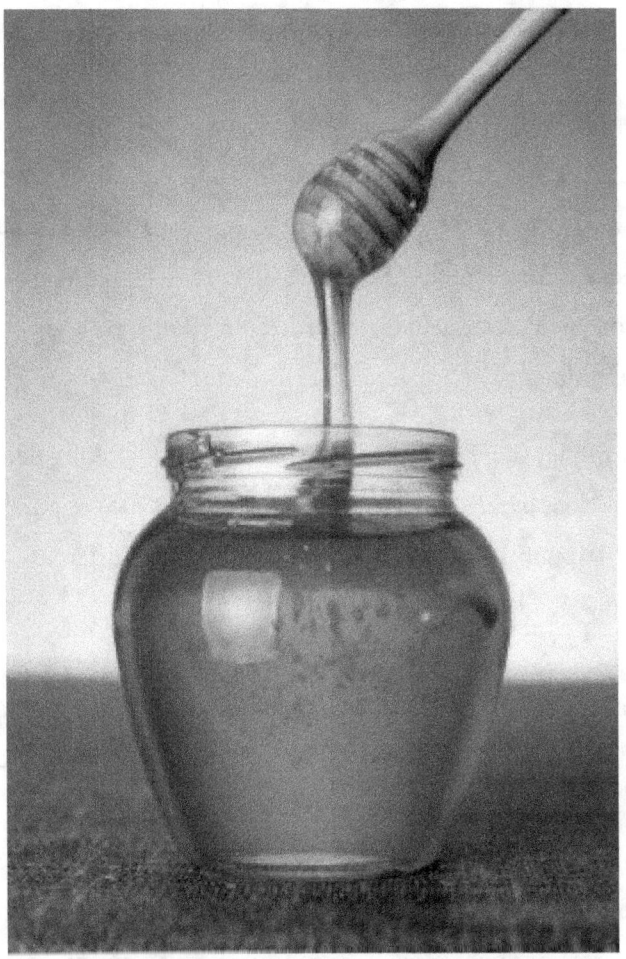

Live Long and Prosper!

Author Bio

Dueep Jyot Singh is a Management and IT Professional who managed to gather Postgraduate qualifications in Management and English and Degrees in Science, French and Education while pursuing different enjoyable career options like being an hospital administrator, IT,SEO and HRD Database Manager/ trainer, movie , radio and TV scriptwriter, theatre artiste and public speaker, lecturer in French, Marketing and Advertising, ex-Editor of Hearts On Fire (now known as Solstice) Books Missouri USA, advice columnist and cartoonist, publisher and Aviation School trainer, ex-moderator on Medico.in, banker, student councilor ,travelogue writer ... among other things!

One fine morning, she decided that she had enough of killing herself by Degrees and went back to her first love -- writing. It's more enjoyable! She already has 48 published academic and 14 fiction- in- different- genre books under her belt.

When she is not designing websites or making Graphic design illustrations for clients , she is browsing through old bookshops hunting for treasures, of which she has an enviable collection – including R.L. Stevenson, O.Henry, Dornford Yates, Maurice Walsh, De Maupassant, Victor Hugo, Sapper, C.N. Williamson, "Bartimeus" and the crown of her collection- Dickens "The Old Curiosity Shop," and "Martin Chuzzlewit" and so on... Just call her "Renaissance Woman") - collecting herbal remedies, acting like Universal Helping Hand/Agony Aunt, or escaping to her dear mountains for a bit of exploring, collecting herbs and plants, and trekking.

Check out some of the other JD-Biz Publishing books

Gardening Series on Amazon

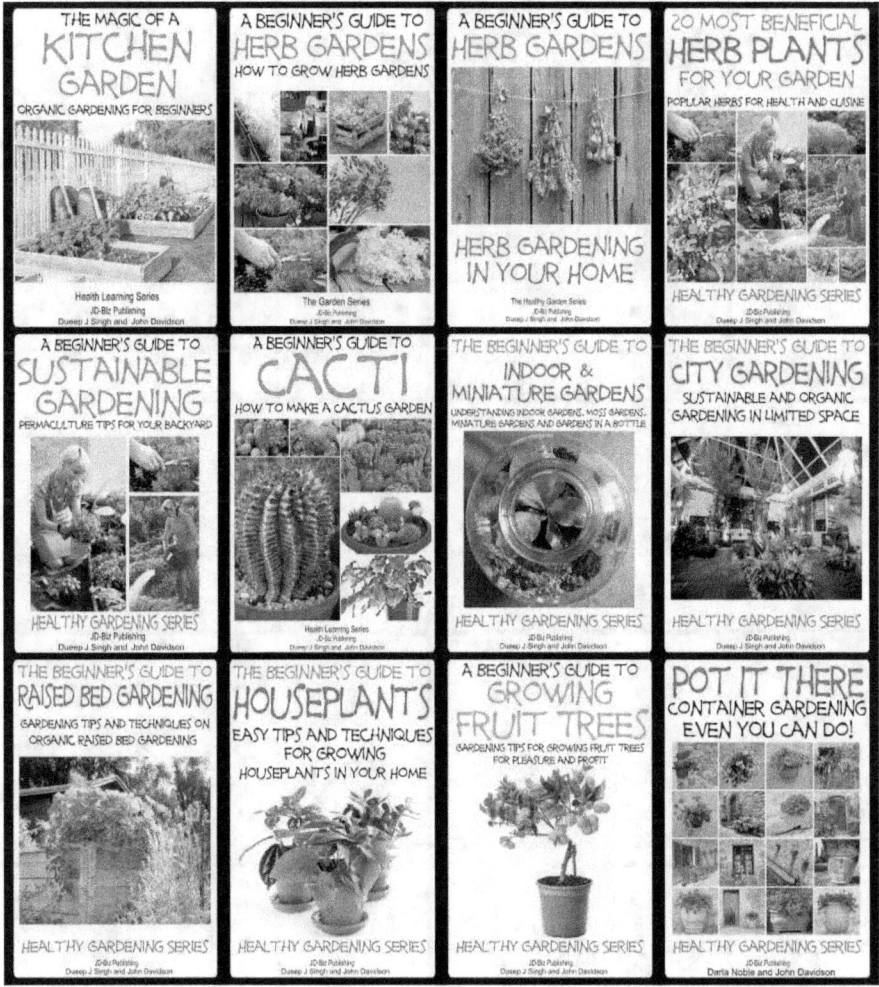

Health Learning Series

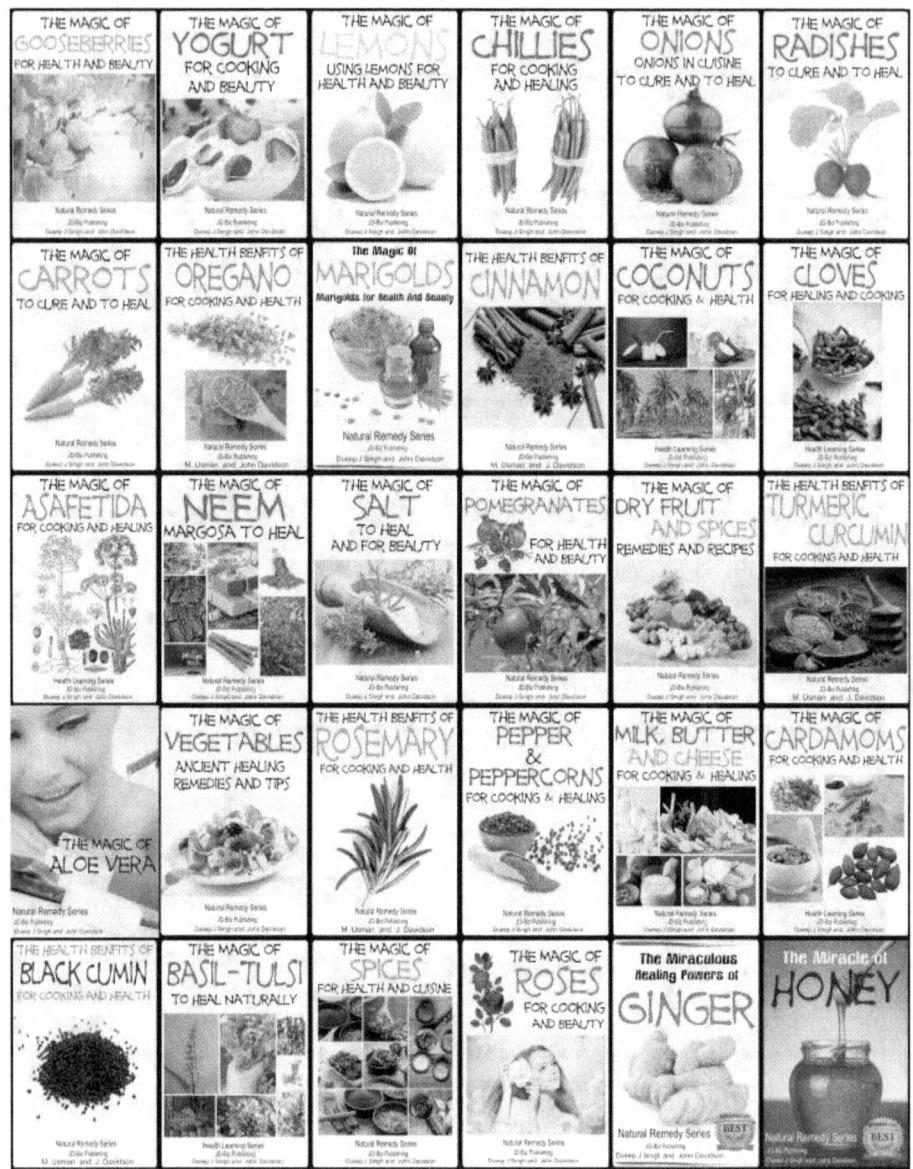

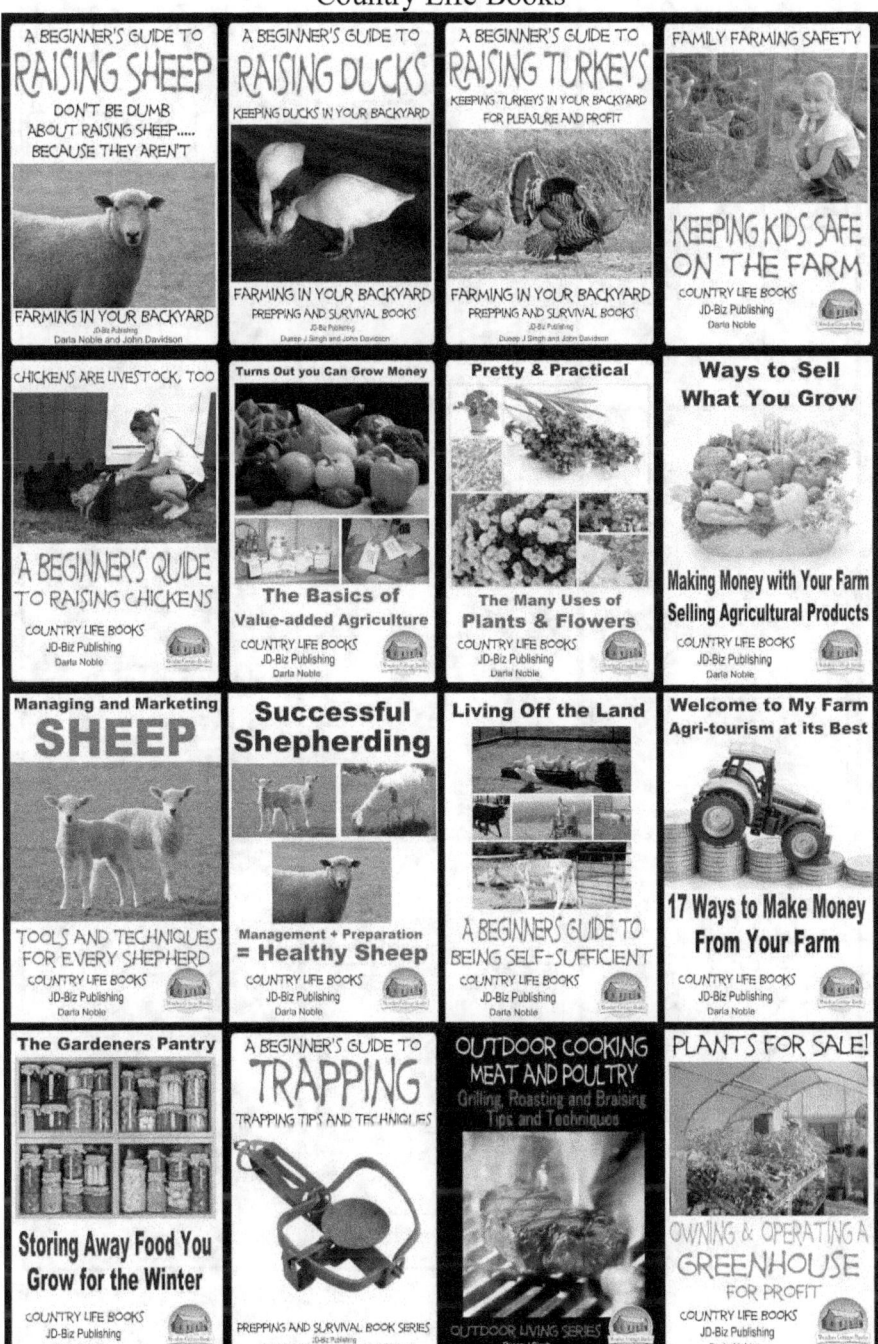

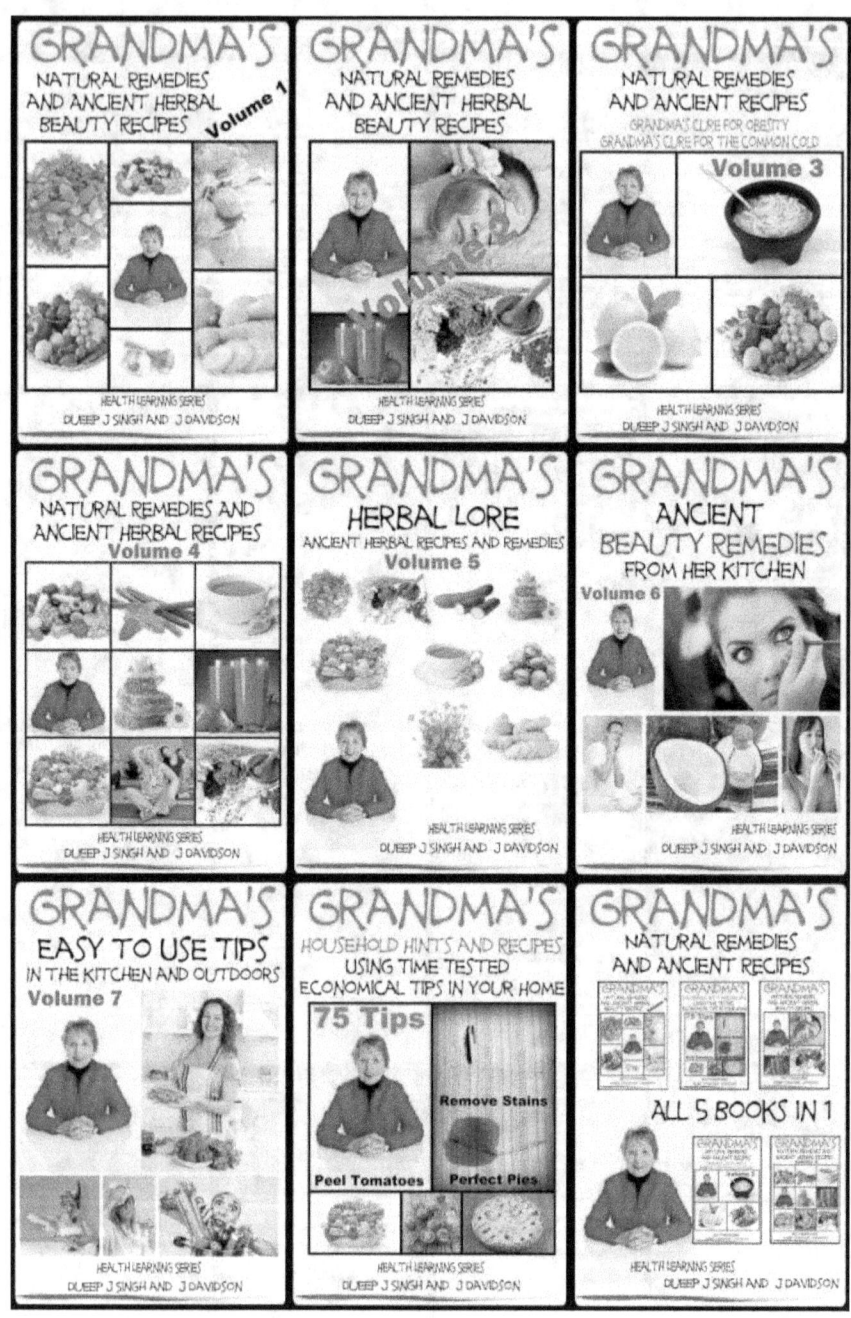

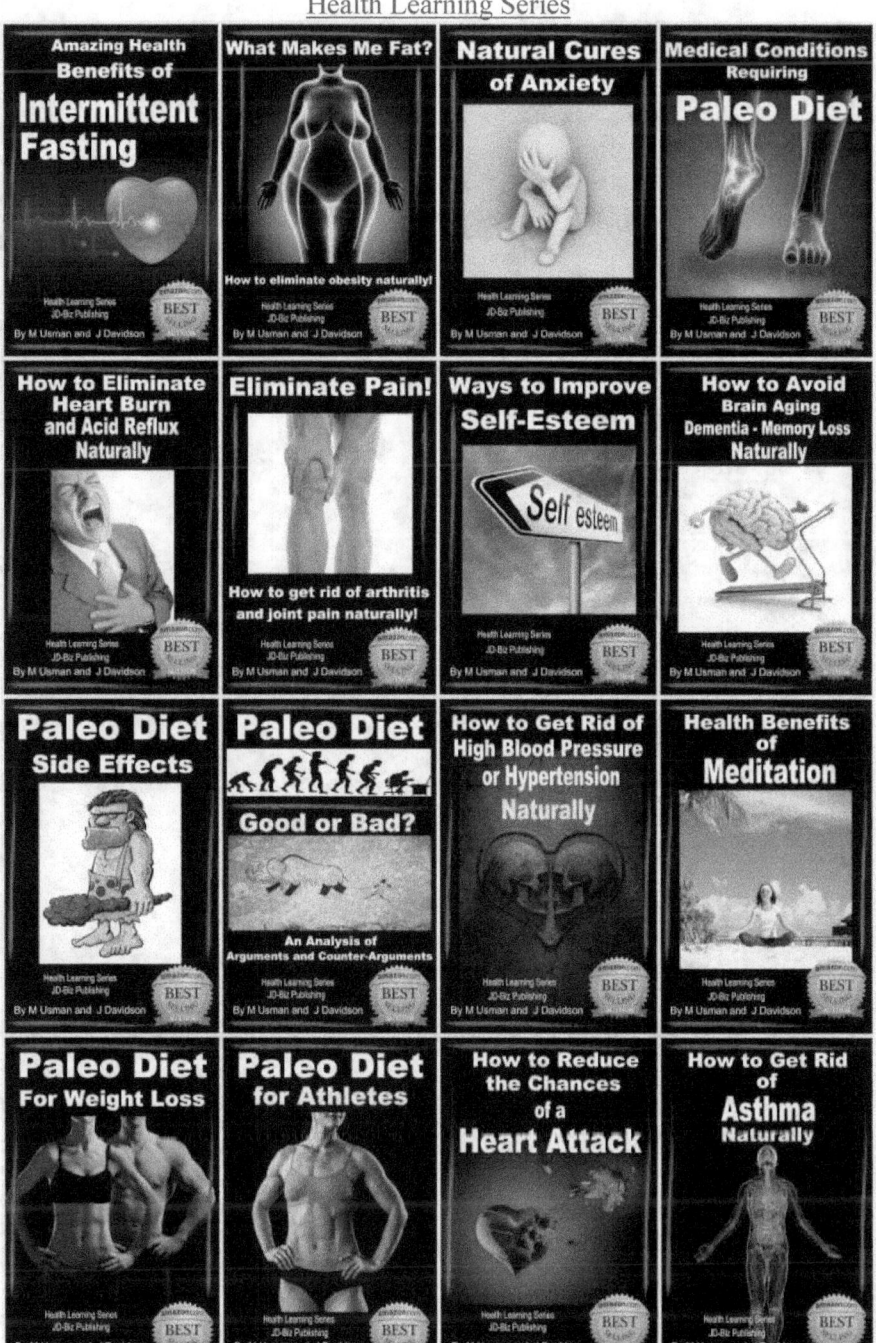

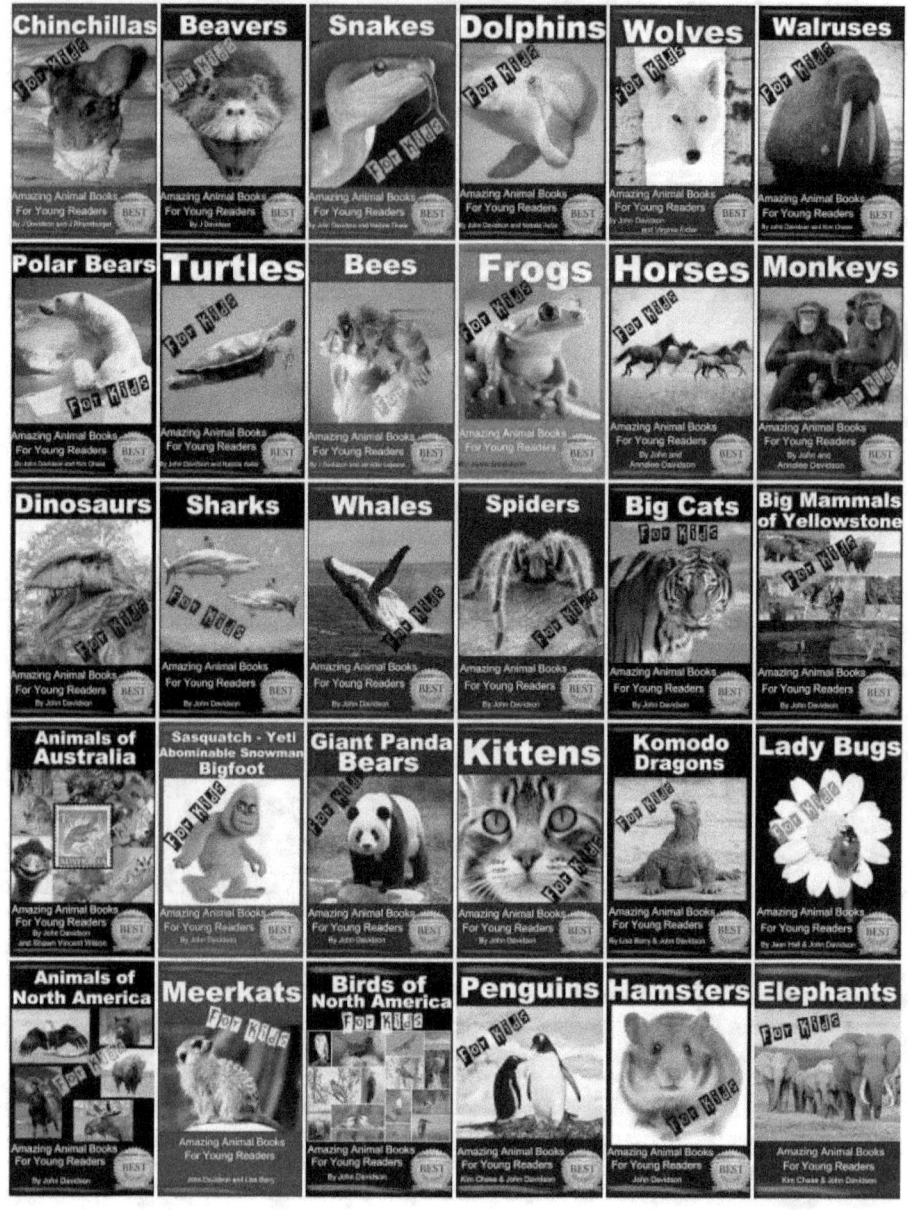

Learn To Draw Series

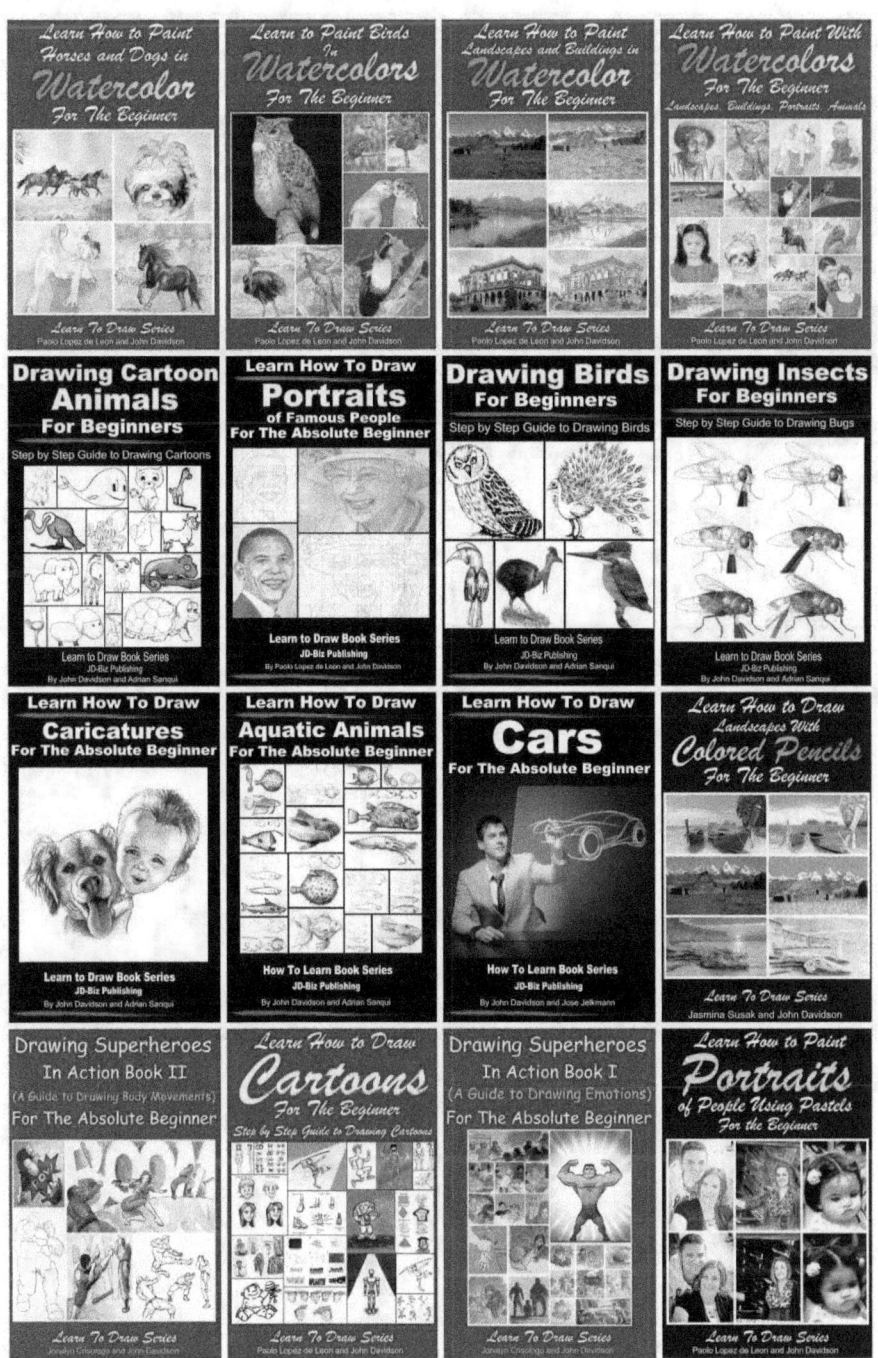

How to Build and Plan Books

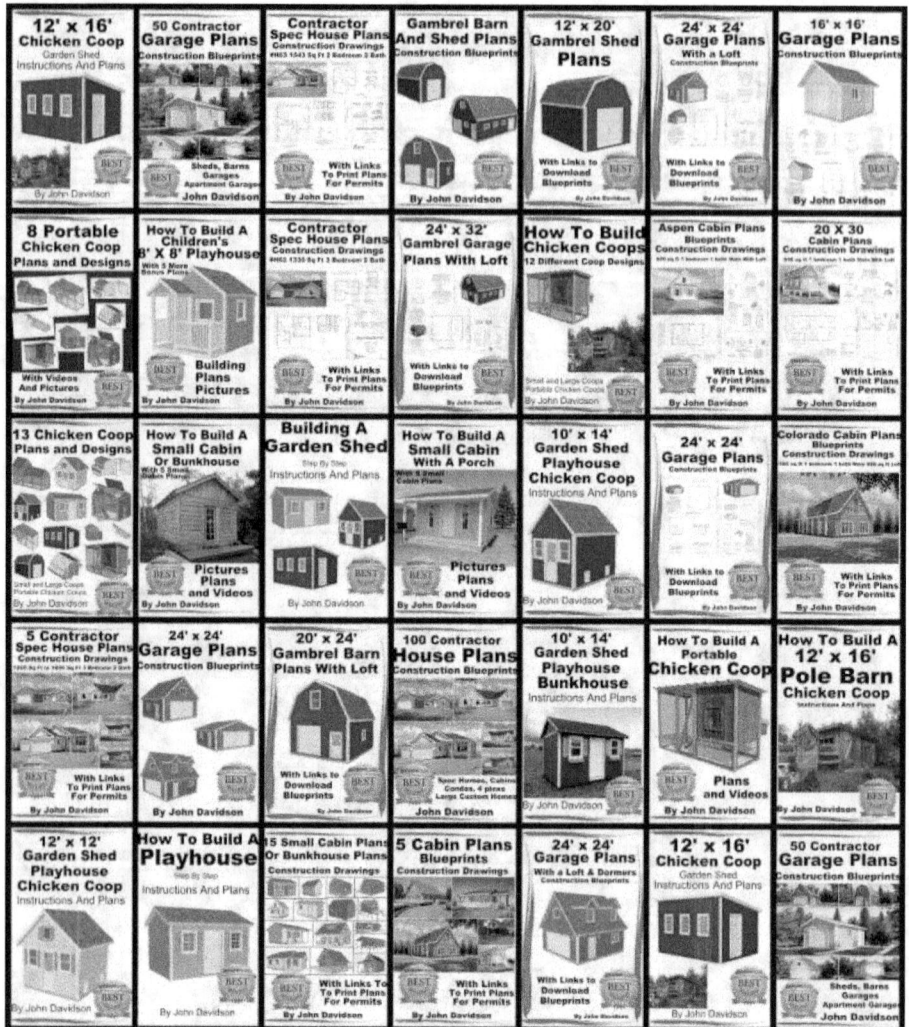

Entrepreneur Book Series

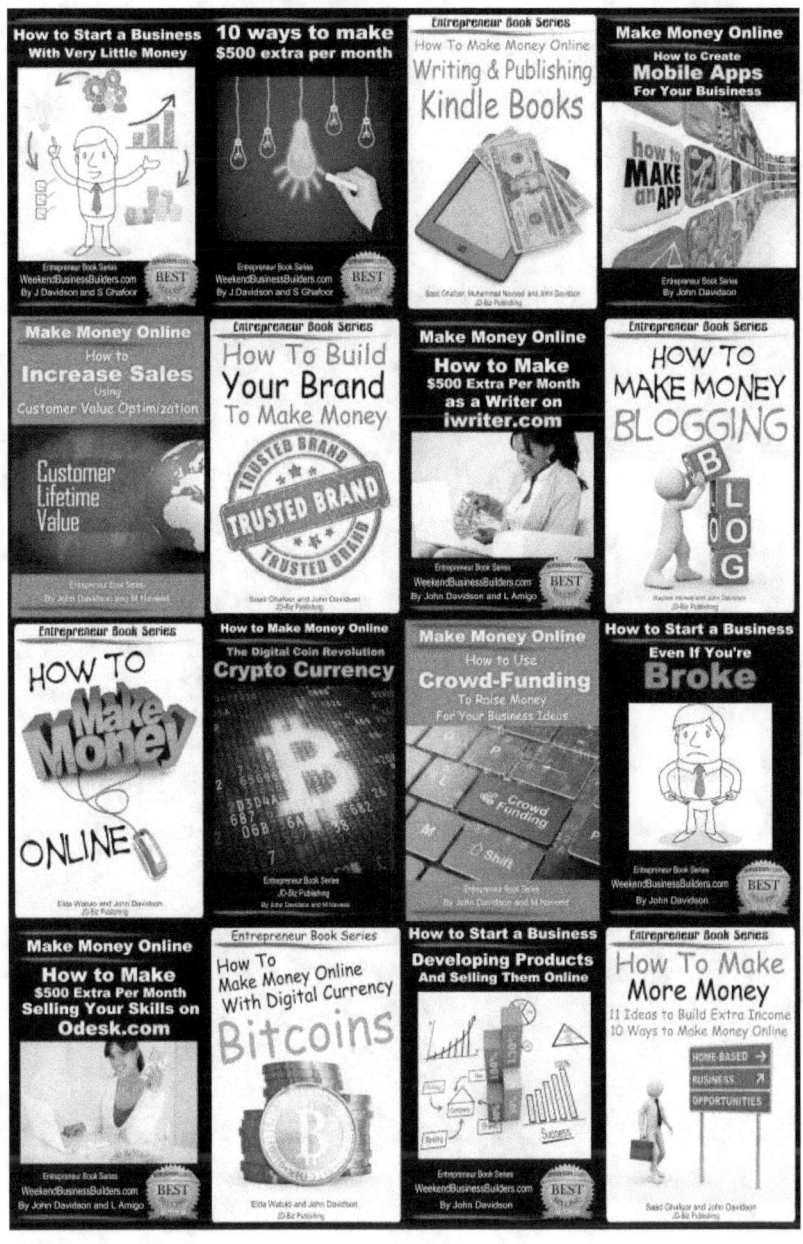

Our books are available at

1. Amazon.com

2. Barnes and Noble

3. Itunes

4. Kobo

5. Smashwords

6. Google Play Books

Download Free Books!

http://MendonCottageBooks.com

Publisher

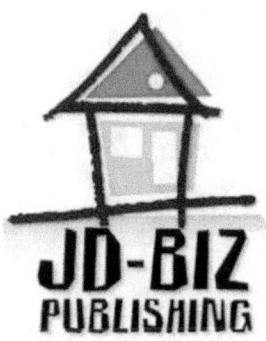

JD-Biz Corp

P O Box 374

Mendon, Utah 84325

http://www.jd-biz.com/

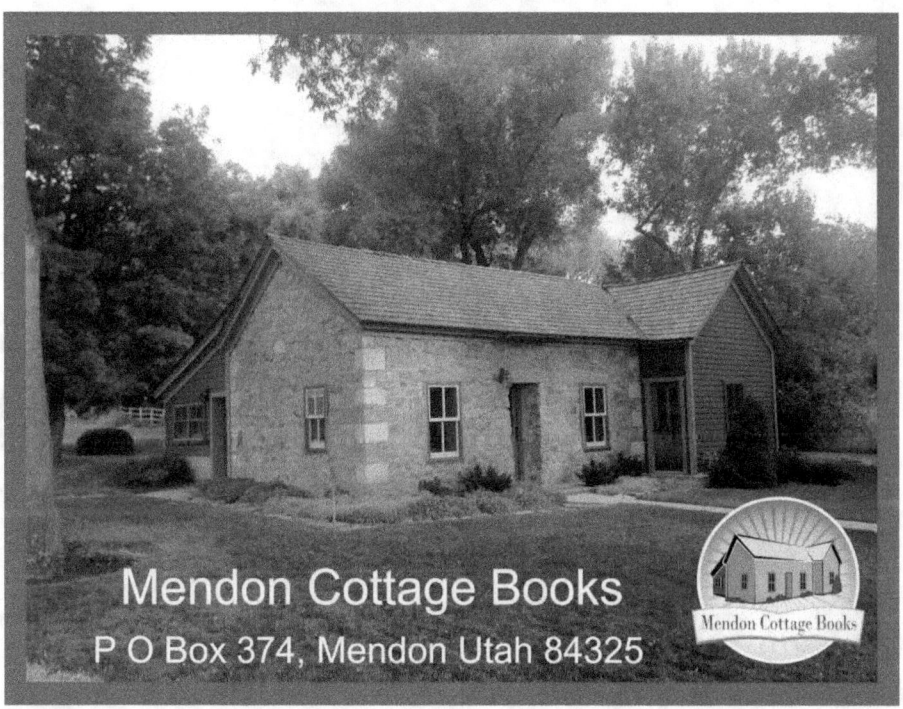